VETERINARIAN BOOK FOR KIDS

How to Become a Vet and Care for Animals

STUART IBORY

TABLE OF CONTENTS

INTRODUCTION

Have you ever wondered what it's like to be a veterinarian? Imagine stepping into a world where your patients range from playful puppies to towering giraffes, where, one moment, you're helping a tiny hamster feel better, and the next, you're figuring out why a lion at the zoo isn't eating. Being a vet is like being a detective, a scientist, and a superhero all rolled into one!

Animals can't tell us when they're feeling sick or what's wrong, so veterinarians must use their knowledge, skills, and even a little creativity to solve medical mysteries. They check for clues— listening to heartbeats, looking at X-rays, and sometimes even peering into an animal's mouth (which is a lot trickier when it belongs to a crocodile!). Vets work in all kinds of places, from busy pet clinics and bustling farms to wildlife reserves deep in the jungle. Some travel the world, helping endangered species, while others develop new medicines to keep animals healthy.

But veterinary medicine isn't just about treating sick animals. It's about preventing illnesses, improving animal lives, and even protecting people. That's right—many diseases can pass between animals and humans, so vets play a big role in keeping everyone safe. Have you ever heard of rabies? Or learned why pets need vaccines? Veterinarians help stop these illnesses before they spread.

The history of veterinary medicine is just as exciting as the work vets do today. For centuries, people have cared for animals, developing remedies and treatments to keep them healthy. As science progressed, so did veterinary medicine, leading to incredible discoveries like X-rays, anesthesia, and advanced surgical techniques. Today, vets use cutting-edge tools and technology that once seemed like science fiction, from robotic-assisted surgeries to DNA testing that helps diagnose rare conditions with precision.

In this book, you'll explore the incredible world of veterinary medicine. You'll learn about the different types of vets, from those who care for pets at home to those who work in wildlife conservation. You'll discover amazing facts about animals, test your knowledge with fun activities, and even try out some hands-on projects to see what it's like to think like a vet. You'll read real-life stories about veterinarians who have saved animals in daring rescues and others who have dedicated their lives to making the world a better place for animals everywhere.

Maybe you already dream of becoming a vet one day, or maybe you just love animals and want to know how to take better care of them. Either way, this book is for you! By the time you finish, you'll understand just how important veterinarians are—and who knows? You might even decide to join their ranks someday.

Now, before you begin your adventure into the world of veterinary medicine, here are a few questions to think about:

- If you could be a vet for any type of animal, which one would you choose and why?

- What do you think would be the most exciting part of being a veterinarian? What might be the hardest part?

- Have you ever helped take care of an animal? How did it make you feel?

- Why do you think veterinarians are important for both animals and people?

- If you could invent a new tool or technology to help vets, what would it be, and how would it work?

Get ready to explore, learn, and be inspired by the amazing world of veterinary medicine!

STUART IBORY

PART 1

EXPLORING THE WORLD OF VETS

CHAPTER 1

What is a Vet?

When animals are in trouble—whether it's a sick puppy, an injured bird, or an elephant with a sore tooth—veterinarians are the ones who step in to help. Vets are animal experts who dedicate their lives to caring for creatures big and small. Their job isn't just about treating illnesses; it's about solving puzzles, showing kindness, and experiencing moments that touch the heart. In this chapter, we'll explore the fascinating world of veterinary medicine and see how vets make a difference every day.

Different Types of Vets

When people think of a veterinarian, they often picture someone who cares for common pets like cats and dogs. While this is an important part of the job, veterinarians actually work with an incredible variety of animals, which can be grouped into five main categories.

Small animal vets are the ones you're most likely to see at local animal clinics. They take care of pets like cats, dogs, rabbits, hamsters, and even fish, focusing on the health and happiness of beloved household companions. Large animal vets, on the other hand, work with farm animals such as cows, horses, and sheep. Their work often takes them to farms and ranches, where they help ensure these animals stay healthy to provide milk, eggs, and other resources.

Wildlife vets dedicate their efforts to animals in the wild, including lions, elephants, and bears. They might work in nature reserves or rescue injured animals, nursing them back to health before releasing them into their natural habitats. Exotic animal vets, meanwhile, specialize in unique pets like snakes, parrots, and lizards. These animals have very different needs compared to typical pets, requiring vets with specialized knowledge and skills.

Finally, zoo vets care for a wide range of animals, from tiny frogs to towering giraffes, ensuring the creatures in zoos remain happy, healthy, and well-cared for.

Each type of veterinarian faces unique challenges, but all share a deep passion for helping animals and making a difference in their lives.

Why Do Animals Need Care?

Just like humans, animals can get sick, injured, or even feel stressed. They need someone who understands their needs and knows how to help them. For example, a dog might have a tummy ache from eating something it shouldn't, or a bird might hurt its wing while flying. Vets step in to figure out what's wrong and find the best way to make them feel better.

Sometimes, animals need care to prevent them from getting sick. Just like we get vaccines to protect us from illnesses, animals need vaccines, too. Vets also help by giving animals regular check-ups to catch any problems early. For example, they might check a cat's teeth to make sure it doesn't have cavities or look at a cow's hooves to ensure they're in good shape.

What Does a Vet Do?

A vet's job is highly hands-on and requires a combination of medical expertise and compassion. Their work involves examining animals, diagnosing health problems, and deciding on the best treatments to keep animals healthy and happy. Regular check-ups are a key part of their role, during which vets assess an animal's overall health by listening to its heartbeat, checking its temperature, and inspecting its fur, feathers, or scales for any signs of concern.

When animals fall ill, vets work to identify the cause of the problem. This often involves taking blood samples, performing X-rays, or using other diagnostic tools to get to the root of the issue. In some cases, their job extends to performing surgeries—whether it's fixing broken bones, removing tumors, or carrying out life-saving operations.

Preventative care is another crucial aspect of a vet's work. Vaccinating animals against diseases helps ensure they stay healthy, and vets play a key role in administering these important shots. Beyond treating animals, vets also educate pet owners on how to care for their companions properly, offering advice on everything from nutrition and grooming to exercise and overall well-being.

Through all these tasks, vets are committed to improving the lives of animals and strengthening the bond between pets and their owners.

The Rewards of Being a Vet

Being a vet can be tough at times. It's not always easy to diagnose problems, and vets sometimes face difficult decisions. However, the rewards are incredible. Imagine the joy of seeing a dog wag its tail again after recovering from surgery or watching a rescued bird fly back into the wild. For vets, these moments make all the hard work worth it.

Vets: Heroes for Animals

Vets are true heroes for animals. They dedicate their lives to understanding and caring for creatures that can't speak for themselves. Whether it's a goldfish with a fin injury or a tiger with a toothache, vets use their skills and knowledge to make a difference. And who knows?

Maybe one day, you could be the hero an animal needs!

Questions

- Imagine you're a vet for a day. What type of vet would you want to be— small animal, large animal, wildlife, exotic, or zoo vet? Why?

- Why do you think animals can't take care of themselves when they are sick or injured? How do vets help them feel better?

- What do you think is the most challenging part of being a vet? What do you think is the most rewarding part?

- If you could help an animal in need, which animal would you choose, and what would you do to help it?

- How are the responsibilities of a vet similar to and different from those of a doctor for humans? Can you think of any tools they might both use?

CHAPTER 2

The History of Veterinary Medicine

The Birth of Veterinary Innovation: X-rays and Beyond

One of the biggest turning points in the history of veterinary medicine came with the invention of X-rays for animals. Imagine a time when doctors couldn't see inside a patient's body. They had to rely on their skills and experience to figure out what was wrong, but that often meant making educated guesses. Then, in 1895, a German scientist named Wilhelm Conrad Roentgen discovered X-rays. It was a game-changer for both human and animal medicine. Suddenly, veterinarians could peer inside an animal's body without having to perform risky surgery. Broken bones, tumors, and foreign objects hidden in an animal's body could be spotted with a simple X-ray. This technology transformed how veterinarians diagnosed and treated animals, and it became an essential part of veterinary practices all over the world.

Vaccines, Antibiotics, and Life-Saving Discoveries

As veterinary medicine advanced, new tools and treatments were developed to help save even more animals. One of the most important discoveries came when scientists realized that diseases could be prevented by using vaccines. In the late 19th century, French scientist Louis Pasteur developed the first rabies vaccine for animals, which had a huge impact on the way veterinarians cared for pets and livestock. Vaccines helped protect animals from diseases like rabies, distemper, and parvovirus, making it easier to keep pets and farm animals healthy. At the same time, the discovery of antibiotics, like penicillin, helped veterinarians fight bacterial infections that once claimed the lives of many animals.

The Rise of Modern Surgery

Surgical techniques have also evolved dramatically over the years. Early surgeries on animals were often rudimentary and risky, with no anesthesia or sterile equipment. But as medical science advanced, so did veterinary surgery. In the early 20th century, veterinarians began to use anesthesia to put animals to sleep during surgery, making procedures less painful and more effective. Surgeons also developed better tools, such as sterilized scalpels and sutures, which made surgeries safer and more successful. Today, veterinarians can perform complex surgeries, like heart transplants or orthopedic procedures, that once seemed impossible.

Meet the Heroes of Veterinary Medicine

While these technological breakthroughs were happening, there were many veterinarians who helped shape the profession through their dedication and passion. One such hero was André-Vincent Pineau, a French veterinarian who is often considered the father of modern veterinary medicine. In the 18th century, Pineau worked tirelessly to improve the care of animals and promote the study of veterinary medicine. He established the first veterinary school in France, which became a model for veterinary education across Europe. Pineau's efforts paved the way for future veterinarians, ensuring that animal care would continue to improve for generations.

Another famous figure in veterinary medicine is James Herriot, a British veterinarian whose stories of working with animals became beloved by millions. Herriot didn't just treat pets in his small town; he also cared for farm animals, working long hours in all kinds of weather. His books, like All Creatures Great and Small, are filled with heartwarming tales of animal care, but they also highlight the challenges veterinarians face. Herriot's dedication to his profession and his compassion for animals made him one of the most famous veterinarians in history.

The Roots of Veterinary Medicine in the U.S.

In the United States, veterinary medicine began to take shape in the 19th century, starting with the establishment of the first veterinary school at the University of Pennsylvania in 1852. Early American veterinarians were often self-taught or trained through apprenticeships, but as the country expanded, so did the need for formal education. By the late 1800s, several more veterinary schools were founded across the U.S., and the profession began to grow. The American Veterinary Medical Association (AVMA), established in 1863, helped to bring veterinarians together and create standards for the profession. Veterinarians in the U.S. played a critical role in improving public health by fighting diseases like tuberculosis, brucellosis, and hoof-and-mouth disease, which had the potential to spread to both animals and humans.

Looking Ahead: The Future of Veterinary Medicine

Today, veterinary medicine continues to evolve with new advancements in technology, treatments, and procedures. Veterinarians can now use cutting-edge tools like ultrasound, MRI machines, and even robotic surgery to help animals. But even with all these modern innovations, the heart of veterinary medicine remains the same: caring for animals, big and small, with compassion and skill. The history of veterinary medicine is filled with remarkable people and inventions, serving as a reminder of the extraordinary contributions veterinarians

have made—and will continue to make—
to the world of animal health.

Questions

- How do you think the invention of X-rays changed the way veterinarians treat animals today? Can you imagine a world without this technology?

- What role do you think veterinarians played in improving public health in the past? How do you think they continue to help protect both animals and humans today?

- If you could meet one famous veterinarian from history, like James Herriot or André-Vincent Pineau, what questions would you ask them about their work and their passion for animal care?

- What are some of the most exciting technological advancements you think we might see in veterinary medicine in the future? How do you think they will change the way we care for animals?

- Why do you think it's important for veterinarians to not only be skilled in medicine but also compassionate toward animals? How do you think empathy helps them do their job better?

CHAPTER 3

A Day in the Life of a Vet

The Morning Begins: Choosing Your First Adventure

It's 7:00 AM, and the clinic is just opening. Today, you're not just reading about a vet—you are the vet. With your stethoscope around your neck and your notebook full of appointments, you step into the busy world of animal care. But wait—what's first on your agenda?

Do you start the day with a routine checkup for a nervous cat named Whiskers or tackle an urgent call about a cow stuck in a muddy ditch?

The Case of Whiskers, the Nervous Cat

If you choose Whiskers, you enter the exam room to find a gray tabby crouched at the far end of the table, her big green eyes watching your every move. Her owner looks worried. "She hasn't been eating much," they explain. You approach Whiskers slowly, speaking softly to keep her calm. But just as you reach out to examine her, she darts under the chair! Uh-oh, it's time to use your skills to coax her out.

After a few moments and a sprinkle of cat treats, Whiskers emerges, and you notice her gums are pale—a sign she might be anemic. You order a blood test, explaining to the owner how important it is to find out what's going on. As you finish the exam, Whiskers lets out a soft "meow" as if to say, "Thanks for being gentle!"

Betsy's Muddy Rescue

If you choose the cow, the phone call is urgent. "Doc, Betsy's stuck in the ditch again!" You jump into your truck and drive out to the farm. When you arrive, you see a very muddy cow looking sheepish in the shallow ditch. With the help of the farmer, you carefully use a harness and a tractor to lift Betsy out. Once she's free, you check her legs for injuries and make sure she's not too stressed. She lets out a loud "moo" as if thanking you for the rescue.

Just as you're packing up to leave, the farmer waves you over. "Doc, while you're here, could you check on the new calf? She hasn't been nursing." The calf's tiny tail wags as you kneel to examine her. You quickly discover she has a sore mouth from teething and reassure the farmer it's nothing serious. A little pain relief, and she'll be back to nursing in no time.

The Afternoon Surge: A Surprising Emergency

The morning has been busy, but the real surprise comes in the afternoon. A family rushes in, cradling their pet parrot, Mango. "He swallowed something shiny!" they exclaim. Sure enough, Mango looks uncomfortable, squawking and fluffing his feathers.

You gently examine him, and with the help of an X-ray, you find the culprit: a shiny earring lodged in his crop. Luckily, you're able to remove it using a special tool, and Mango quickly perks up. "Good as new," you tell the family as Mango whistles happily, clearly back to his usual self.

Ending the Day with Reflection

As the sun begins to set, you look back on a day filled with unexpected challenges, clever problem-solving, and moments of pure joy. From calming a nervous cat to rescuing a muddy cow to helping a mischievous parrot, your work has made a big difference in the lives of both animals and their humans.

Veterinarians face new surprises every day, and the job takes patience, creativity, and a whole lot of heart. Whether it's a routine checkup or an emergency, every moment is an opportunity to help an animal in need.

Questions

- How would you have handled Whiskers' nervousness during her exam? What techniques would you use to keep an animal calm?

- What do you think is the most challenging part of being a veterinarian, and how would you handle it?

- If you were called to help an animal stuck in a tricky situation, like Betsy the cow, what tools or skills do you think you would need?

- Why do you think it's important for veterinarians to work closely with pet owners or farmers? How does teamwork help solve problems?

- Which case in today's adventure was your favorite, and why? Can you imagine yourself solving a similar problem in real life?

CHAPTER 4

The Tools of the Trade

What's Inside a Vet's Toolbox?

Every veterinarian has a special toolbox filled with tools that help them take care of animals. Some tools are easy to recognize, like a stethoscope, while others might surprise you. Imagine you're holding a stethoscope right now. You place the flat part on your dog's chest and listen carefully. What do you hear? That's the sound of their heartbeat—a steady "lub-dub, lub-dub." Vets use this tool to check if an animal's heart and lungs are healthy. But did you know a stethoscope can also help detect purring in cats? A loud purr can make it tricky to hear their heartbeat, which can turn a checkup into a game of patience and listening skills.

Now, let's say you pick up a small flashlight-like tool called an otoscope. What do you think it's for? You might guess it's for shining light into dark spaces—and you'd be right! But instead of lighting up a room, vets use an otoscope to peek inside animals' ears. An otoscope can reveal ear infections, pesky mites, or even a tiny ball of dirt stuck inside a curious puppy's ear.

Tools for Big and Small Jobs

Not all veterinary tools fit neatly into a bag or pocket. Some are tiny, like bird-sized splints, which are delicate supports for a bird's broken leg or wing. Picture this: A small parakeet named Sunny has a mishap and hurts her leg. The vet uses a tiny splint, no bigger than a toothpick, to help her heal. It might seem unusual to make such small tools, but vets care for animals of all sizes, and that means being prepared for anything.

On the other hand, there are tools designed for very big jobs. For instance, imagine a large scale that is big enough to weigh an elephant at the zoo. Vets use these giant scales to track the health of massive animals like elephants, giraffes, and rhinos. Keeping track of their weight helps vets know if they're eating enough or if something might be wrong. It's not just about the tools—it's about adapting them to the patient's size.

Unusual Tools for Unusual Animals

Sometimes, veterinarians use tools you might never expect. For example, have you ever heard of a snake hook? This tool is a long, curved rod that helps vets handle snakes safely, keeping both the vet and the snake calm and secure. Or what about a special fish anesthesia system? Yes, that's a real thing! Vets use it to gently sedate fish so they can perform surgeries or remove hooks from a fish's mouth without causing stress.

Another interesting tool is a dental float. This isn't a float like you'd use in a swimming pool—it's a file used to smooth out a horse's teeth. Horses' teeth grow continuously, and if they get too sharp, it can make eating painful. The dental float helps ensure the horse's teeth are smooth and comfortable.

Create Your Own Mini Vet Kit

Here's something fun you can do at home: create your mini vet kit! You can start with safe household items. For example, a toy stethoscope can help you imagine listening to a pet's heartbeat, while a flashlight can act as your otoscope. Cotton balls can stand in for bandage wraps, and a notebook can be your medical chart for recording "patient" information. You don't need fancy tools to practice imagining yourself as a vet. The important thing is to think about how tools are used to help animals feel better.

The Heart Behind the Tools

No matter how advanced or unusual the tools are, what matters most is how they're used—with care, patience, and creativity. Every tool in a vet's toolbox has a purpose, whether it's helping a tiny bird, a towering giraffe, or a beloved family pet. As you explore these tools, remember that they're more than just objects—they're a way to connect with animals and make a difference in their lives.

Questions

- Which tool from the chapter do you find most interesting, and why do you think it's important for animal care?

- If you were designing a new tool to help animals, what would it do, and how would it work?

- Why do you think it's important for veterinarians to have tools that work for both tiny animals like birds and big ones like elephants?

- Can you think of a situation where a vet might need to invent a creative solution using the tools they already have?

- If you made your mini vet kit, what items would you include, and how would you use them to help animals?

CHAPTER 5

Skills Every Vet Needs

The Eyes of a Detective: Observation Skills

Being a veterinarian is a lot like being a detective. Animals can't tell you how they feel, so it's up to vets to notice the little clues that reveal what's wrong. Imagine walking into a barn where a horse named Daisy stands quietly. At first, she looks fine. But when you look closer, you notice she's not eating her hay, her ears are drooping, and she's shifting her weight uncomfortably. These are small signs, but to a vet, they're a big deal.

Let's try an activity! Look at the photos or imagine different scenarios: a dog scratching its ears nonstop, a cat that's stopped purring, or a parrot fluffed up in the corner of its cage. Can you spot what might be wrong? Vets use their keen observation skills to figure out if an animal is sick, injured, or just having a bad day.

A Heart Full of Empathy

When a scared puppy is trembling in the exam room or a family is worried about their beloved sheep, empathy becomes a vet's most powerful skill. Empathy means understanding and caring about what others feel, whether it's the wagging tail of a dog saying thank you or a worried glance from an owner.

One inspiring story is about a vet who worked with a nervous rescue dog named Bella. Bella was terrified of people and would hide every time someone approached. Instead of rushing, the vet spent weeks sitting quietly near Bella, letting her get used to the presence of a kind human. Slowly but surely, Bella began to trust again, and her transformation into a happy, playful dog brought tears to her owner's eyes.

Teamwork Saves the Day

Vets don't work alone—they rely on a team of dedicated people, including vet techs, nurses, and even pet owners. Take the story of a sea turtle named Shelly who had swallowed a fishing hook. Removing the hook required careful coordination: one person gently held Shelly's flippers to keep her calm, another monitored her breathing, and the vet performed a delicate procedure to remove the hook. Without teamwork, Shelly's recovery wouldn't have been possible.

Teamwork doesn't stop at the clinic, either. Sometimes, vets partner with wildlife organizations, farmers, or even police officers to protect animals and keep them healthy. Whether it's rescuing a stranded dolphin or helping a farmer care for a herd of sheep, working together makes a huge difference.

Thinking Outside the Box: Problem-Solving Skills

Sometimes, being a vet means solving problems no one has faced before. For example, a vet in a snowy town once had to figure out how to save a goose that got stuck in an icy pond. Using quick thinking, the vet crafted a floating platform to safely reach the goose without falling in.

Problem-solving can also mean inventing new tools. One vet created special boots for a dog named Max, who had trouble walking on slippery floors. With some creativity and determination, the vet turned an everyday challenge into a happy solution for Max and his family.

The Real Superpower: Combining It All

Observation, empathy, teamwork, and problem-solving don't work alone. A great vet combines these skills to give every animal the best care possible. Imagine being a vet who notices a rabbit isn't eating, understands the owner's worry, teams up with a colleague to perform a safe exam, and comes up with a clever way to help the rabbit recover. Every skill builds on the others, creating a superpower that saves lives.

Questions

- Why do you think observation is one of the most important skills a vet needs? Can you think of a time you noticed something others didn't?

- How does empathy help a vet connect with both animals and their owners? Why do you think this skill is so important?

- What's an example of teamwork you've seen or been a part of? How do you think teamwork helps vets in their daily work?

- Imagine you're a vet faced with a problem you've never seen before, like the icy pond goose or Max's slippery floor issue. What creative solution might you try?

- If you could practice one of these skills right now—observation, empathy, teamwork, or problem-solving—which one would you choose, and how would you use it?

PART 2

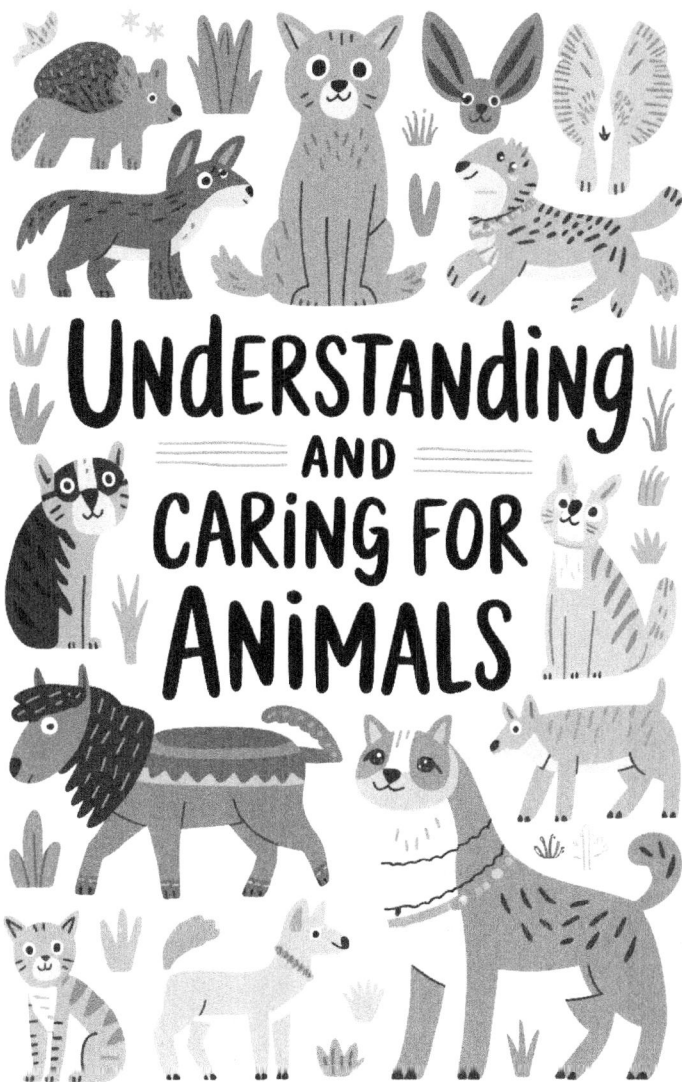

Understanding AND CARING FOR ANIMALS

CHAPTER 6

Understanding Animal Behavior

Animals speak their own unique language, and as a future vet, it's your job to learn how to understand it! Whether it's a happy dog wagging its tail or a grumpy cat flicking its ears, every action tells a story. In this chapter, we'll dive into the fascinating world of animal behavior and learn how to decode what our furry, feathered, and scaly friends are trying to say.

Why Understanding Behavior Matters

Imagine you're a detective, and your case is figuring out why a dog won't eat or why a bird keeps flapping its wings wildly. Animals can't talk like humans, but they communicate in their own ways. By observing their behavior, vets can uncover clues about their health, happiness, or even fears. Understanding animal behavior is a superpower that helps you build trust with animals and give them the care they need.

Body Language Basics

Animals often communicate through their body language, using their movements and postures to express their feelings. For example, dogs commonly wag their tails to show happiness, but the speed and direction of the wag can tell you even more. A slow wag may indicate uncertainty, while a fast, wide wag is a sign of excitement. If a dog tucks its tail between its legs, it could be feeling scared or anxious.

Cats also use their tails to communicate. A tail held high often signals confidence, while a twitching tail may mean the cat is annoyed or agitated. If a cat flattens its ears or hisses, it's a clear warning to stay back, as it's likely feeling threatened.

Birds use their feathers to express various emotions. When birds fluff up their feathers, they're either trying to stay warm or showing that they're relaxed. However, if they remain puffed up for an extended period, it could indicate that they're unwell. A bird that bobs its head up and down may be showing excitement or hunger.

Horses, too, communicate a lot with their ears. When a horse's ears are facing forward, it's a sign that the horse is curious or interested in something. On the other hand, when a horse pins its ears back, it usually means it's feeling angry or uncomfortable. If a horse starts stomping its hooves, it might be showing impatience or irritation.

Vocal Clues

Animals also communicate through sounds, each noise carrying its own meaning. Dogs, for example, use barking to express themselves in different ways. A playful bark is often lively and high-pitched, while an alarm bark is more urgent and intense. Whining is another common sound dogs make, which can signal that they are anxious or need something, like attention or food.

Cats primarily use purring to communicate contentment, but this sound can also occur when they are in pain. In these cases, the purring acts as a way for the cat to soothe itself. Pay attention to the context of the purring to understand if they are comfortable or in distress.

Birds are known for their singing, which is typically a sign that they are happy or content. However, if a bird starts squawking, it could indicate stress or an attempt to warn others of a threat in their environment. The tone and frequency of these vocalizations can give important clues about how the bird is feeling.

Behavior in Different Settings

Animals often behave differently depending on their environment. A dog, for example, might be calm and playful at home, but at the vet clinic, it could become nervous or fearful. As a vet, it's crucial to understand how different settings influence animal behavior and to adjust your approach to make them feel as comfortable as possible.

Gentle movements and a soothing voice can be very effective in helping a nervous animal feel safe. When handling a frightened cat, it's important to provide a quiet, sheltered space where the cat can hide during an exam, helping it feel more secure. Additionally, approaching animals at their eye level instead of towering over them can prevent feelings of intimidation, making them more at ease during interactions. Recognizing and responding to these behaviors ensures that animals are treated with care and respect, no matter where they are.

Interactive Activity: Decode the Behavior!

Let's put your detective skills to the test! Below are some scenarios. Can you guess what the animal is trying to tell you?

- A dog is barking and wagging its tail, but its ears are pinned back.

  - What it means: The dog might be feeling conflicted—excited but also nervous.

- A cat is lying on its side, showing its belly but swishing its tail back and forth.

  - What it means: The cat might seem relaxed, but the tail swish is a warning to stay away.

- A bird flaps its wings and chirps loudly when you approach its cage.

  - What it means: The bird is likely excited and happy to see you!

Building Trust Through Understanding

Understanding animal behavior is not only about solving problems but also about building trust. When animals feel safe, they are more likely to cooperate with you. To earn their trust, patience is key. Rushing an animal into doing something they're uncomfortable with can make them anxious or frightened. Instead, give them time to adjust and feel at ease.

Rewarding good behavior is another effective way to build trust. Treats and praise help animals associate positive experiences with their interactions with you, making them more willing to cooperate in the future. It's also important to learn the animal's preferences—some may enjoy belly rubs, while others prefer a gentle scratch behind the ears. By paying attention to what they enjoy, you can create a bond based on mutual respect and understanding.

Amazing Animal Behavior Facts

Did you know that dogs can sense your emotions? They have an incredible ability to detect how you're feeling and will often try to comfort you if you're sad or upset. It's one of the reasons why dogs are such great companions.

Cats also have a unique way of showing affection. They use something called the "slow blink" to communicate trust. If a cat looks at you and blinks slowly, it's their way of saying that they feel safe and comfortable around you.

Octopuses are another amazing example of animal intelligence. These clever creatures can solve puzzles and even open jars! With their incredible problem-solving skills, they are considered some of the smartest animals in the ocean.

Becoming a Behavior Expert

If you're passionate about understanding animals, you can specialize in animal behavior when you become a vet. Behavior specialists help animals with issues like anxiety or aggression, making life better for both pets and their owners. Who knows? One day, you could help a nervous puppy become a confident dog or teach a parrot to stop biting!

Understanding animal behavior is like learning a secret language. The more you observe, the better you'll get at understanding what animals are saying. So, grab a notebook and start practicing by watching the animals around you. You'll be amazed at how much they have to say!

Questions

- Why do you think it's important for a vet to understand animal behavior when diagnosing health problems?

- How can a vet's knowledge of body language and vocal clues help build trust with animals?

- What are some ways you could help an anxious pet feel more comfortable during a visit to the vet?

- How would you approach a situation where an animal is showing conflicting signals, like a dog that's excited but also nervous?

- If you could specialize in animal behavior, what kind of problems would you want to help animals with, and why?

CHAPTER 7

Amazing Animal Facts

Animals are full of surprises, and the more you learn about them, the more fascinating they become. Whether it's a common pet like a dog or a mysterious creature from the wild, every animal has unique abilities that make them extraordinary. In this chapter, we'll uncover some surprising facts, dive into a fun, hands-on experiment, and challenge your curiosity with animal mysteries. Get ready to explore the incredible world of animals like a true vet!

Did You Know?

Dogs have a superpower that sets them apart: their sense of smell is up to 100,000 times stronger than a human's. This incredible ability allows them to sniff out things we can't even imagine. They can detect a drop of liquid in an Olympic-sized pool, identify people by their scent alone, and even help doctors diagnose illnesses like cancer or diabetes. Some dogs are trained to locate missing people or sniff out explosives, making their noses one of the most powerful tools in the animal kingdom.

Here's a fun experiment to understand how a dog's nose works: create your own "smell test." Gather items with distinct scents, like cinnamon, vanilla extract, or lemon juice. Place them on cotton balls and hide them in different areas of a room. Then, close your eyes and try to find them using only your nose. It's harder than you think! Imagine how much more amazing it would be if your sense of smell were as strong as a dog's.

Animal Curiosities

Some animals have abilities that seem almost magical. Did you know that the koala is one of the sleepiest creatures on Earth? These cuddly marsupials from Australia can sleep up to 22 hours a day. Why so much snoozing? Digesting eucalyptus leaves, their favorite (and only) food, takes a lot of energy, so they need extra rest.

If you thought the cheetah was the fastest animal, think again! The peregrine falcon holds the record for speed, diving at over 240 miles per hour to catch its prey. Meanwhile, blue whales are the loudest animals on Earth, producing sounds louder than a jet engine. Their calls can travel across hundreds of miles underwater, helping them communicate in the vast ocean.

And here's something truly mind-boggling: octopuses have three hearts! Two pump blood to their gills, while the third pumps blood to the rest of their body. Interestingly, the heart that supplies the body stops beating when the octopus swims. This unique adaptation allows these clever creatures to thrive in their underwater habitats.

Encouraging Curiosity

Now it's your turn to explore. Let's try a "fact challenge" to test what you've learned. Can you guess which animal can regrow its limbs? If you guessed "starfish," you're correct! These fascinating sea creatures can regenerate an arm if they lose one—and some can even grow a whole new body from just one arm.

Fact challenges are a great way to stay curious. You can make your own by looking up surprising animal abilities and quizzing your friends and family. For example, which animal has the best eyesight (the eagle) or which one never sleeps (the bullfrog)? You'll find there's always something new and exciting to discover.

Why These Facts Matter

Amazing animal facts aren't just fun—they help us understand and appreciate the creatures we share the planet with. Every unique ability serves a purpose, whether it's a dog's sense of smell, a falcon's speed, or a whale's booming call. Learning about these traits can spark deeper questions: How did these abilities evolve? How do they help animals survive? This kind of curiosity is essential for vets, who need to understand animals' unique needs to care for them effectively.

When you watch a bird fly, a dog sniff, or a cat nap, try to imagine what's happening behind the scenes. Every behavior has a story, and every animal has something incredible to teach us. By paying attention to these details, you'll start to see animals in a whole new way—like a real animal behavior expert.

Questions

- Why do you think some animals have such extreme abilities, like a falcon's speed or a whale's loud calls?

- How could understanding an animal's unique traits help a vet provide better care?

- If you could spend a day with any animal mentioned in this chapter, which one would it be and why?

- What was the most surprising fact you learned? Did it make you more curious about that animal?

- Can you think of an animal with an amazing ability not mentioned here? What makes it special?

CHAPTER 8

How to Care for Pets

Being a great pet owner is about more than giving belly rubs or sharing snacks— it's about taking responsibility for your pet's health and happiness. As a future vet, understanding pet care is a vital skill. Whether it's feeding schedules, exercise routines, or knowing how to handle emergencies, good pet care starts with knowledge and preparation.

Daily Pet Care: A Vet's Perspective

A vet's advice always begins with the basics: a healthy diet, plenty of exercise, and lots of love. Each animal has its own needs. For example, dogs thrive on consistent feeding schedules with nutritious food that supports their energy levels, while cats need a diet rich in protein. Animals like sheep require grazing space and regular hoof care, and they can benefit from check-ups to prevent common conditions like foot rot.

By learning about these unique needs, you'll not only become a better pet owner but also gain insight into what vets evaluate during check-ups. They look for signs of health issues related to poor nutrition or lack of exercise and guide pet owners in making improvements.

Creating Happy, Healthy Habits

Exercise isn't just fun—it's essential. Pets like dogs need daily walks to stay fit, both physically and mentally. Sheep enjoy opportunities to roam and graze, which supports their natural instincts. Cats might not need walks, but interactive toys and climbing structures are great ways to keep them active indoors. When animals get enough physical activity, they're less likely to develop health problems, and as a vet, you'll help pet owners understand this connection.

Proper grooming is another important habit. Brushing your pet's fur, cleaning their ears, and trimming their nails aren't just for appearances—they help prevent issues like skin infections or overgrown nails, which can cause pain. Vets often teach pet owners how to handle grooming and monitor for signs of discomfort, making the experience easier for everyone involved.

Be Prepared: Pet First Aid

Even the healthiest pets can have accidents, so it's important to know what to do in an emergency. Imagine your dog steps on a sharp object during a hike or your sheep injures its leg while grazing. Having a pet first-aid kit can make a big difference. Include bandages, antiseptic wipes, and a pet-safe thermometer. Learning how to check your pet's pulse or clean a small wound is something every aspiring vet can practice.

Veterinarians often host workshops for pet owners, teaching them basic first-aid skills. By participating, you not only learn valuable lessons but also get a glimpse into the hands-on aspect of veterinary work. These skills save lives and strengthen the bond between you and your pet.

Kid Hero Stories: Caring Like a Vet

Let's meet some inspiring kids who took pet care to the next level. Emily, an 11-year-old, noticed her sheep limping one day. Instead of ignoring it, she carefully checked its hooves and discovered a small stone lodged between them. She removed it gently and then called her vet to ensure everything was okay.

Another hero, Max, set up a neighborhood dog-walking service, helping busy pet owners give their dogs the exercise they needed. Max even started learning about dog breeds to understand their specific needs better, a skill that will come in handy when he becomes a vet.

These stories show how everyday actions can make a big difference in an animal's life. By thinking like a vet, you can spot problems early and find solutions that keep pets healthy and happy.

Becoming a Pet Care Expert

As you practice caring for pets, you're building skills that veterinarians use every day. Observing your pet's behavior, maintaining their health, and being prepared for emergencies are all steps toward becoming an animal care expert. Who knows? The lessons you learn now could inspire you to help even more animals as a vet in the future.

Questions

- What are three daily habits you can practice to improve your pet's health?

- How can exercise prevent health issues in pets, and why is this important to a vet's work?

- What would you include in your own pet first-aid kit, and how would you use it in an emergency?

- How do grooming routines help pets stay healthy, and what might a vet look for during grooming?

- What did you learn from Emily and Max's stories that you can apply to your own experiences with animals?

CHAPTER 9

Exotic Animals and Their Special Care

Exotic animals are some of the most fascinating creatures to care for, but they also bring unique challenges to the veterinary world. From reptiles to birds and even small mammals like hedgehogs, these animals often need specialized care that goes beyond what you'd do for a dog or cat. Becoming a vet who treats exotic animals is like entering a world full of puzzles, where you solve mysteries about diet, habitat, and behavior to keep these incredible creatures healthy and happy.

Understanding the Needs of Exotic Pets

Unlike traditional pets, exotic animals have very specific needs that mimic their natural habitats. Reptiles like snakes and lizards require carefully controlled temperatures and humidity levels to thrive. A bearded dragon, for example, needs a basking area to stay warm and a UVB light to absorb calcium and keep its bones strong. Without these conditions, reptiles can develop serious health problems.

Birds, too, present unique challenges. Parrots, for instance, are highly social and intelligent animals that need mental stimulation and a proper diet to stay healthy. Feeding them only seeds might seem okay, but it can actually lead to malnutrition. Parrots thrive on a variety of fruits, vegetables, and specially formulated pellets.

Small mammals like hedgehogs and sugar gliders also need careful attention.

Hedgehogs require a balanced diet and a safe, quiet environment to avoid stress, while sugar gliders need plenty of social interaction and space to glide. Vets who care for exotic animals need to know about these unique requirements and educate pet owners to provide the right care.

Stories from the Exotic Side of Vet Work

Every vet who treats exotic animals has memorable stories to tell. Dr. Harper, for example, once cared for a sick chameleon named Ziggy. Ziggy wasn't eating, and his vibrant green color had turned dull. After a thorough examination, Dr. Harper discovered that Ziggy's enclosure wasn't warm enough, and he wasn't getting enough UVB light. Dr. Harper worked with Ziggy's owner to redesign his habitat, and soon, Ziggy was back to climbing branches and showing off his bright colors.

Then there's Dr. Lee, who treated a macaw named Mango. Mango had started plucking out her feathers—a sign of stress. Dr. Lee found out that Mango's cage was too small, and she didn't have enough toys to keep her entertained. Dr. Lee helped Mango's owner create a more enriching environment, and Mango's feathers grew back as her mood improved.

These stories highlight the detective work involved in exotic animal care. Vets don't just treat symptoms; they investigate the root causes, which often tie back to the animal's environment or diet.

Design Your Dream Exotic Animal Clinic

Caring for exotic animals often requires special equipment and setups. Imagine designing your very own exotic animal clinic. What would it look like? Perhaps you'd have special rooms for reptiles with adjustable heat lamps and misting systems to create the perfect conditions. Your bird care area could feature a soundproof aviary for stressed parrots, and you might include a small mammal section with climbing spaces for sugar gliders.

Think about what tools you'd need, like tiny X-ray machines for snakes or an incubator for baby turtles. A clinic like this would be an amazing place for exotic animals to get the care they need while teaching pet owners how to care for their unique companions.

Becoming an Expert in the Unusual

Exotic animal care is a growing field in veterinary medicine. These animals are often misunderstood, which means vets who specialize in them play a crucial role in educating pet owners. If you love the idea of working with creatures like parrots, snakes, or hedgehogs, you could one day become a specialist in exotic animal medicine. It's a career path that combines science, creativity, and a passion for the extraordinary.

Questions

- What are some of the unique challenges exotic animals face in captivity, and how can vets help solve them?

- Why is it important to recreate an exotic animal's natural habitat when caring for them?

- How do stories like Ziggy the chameleon or Mango, the Macaw show the problem-solving skills that vets need?

- If you were designing an exotic animal clinic, what features would you include to make it a safe and comfortable space?

- What excites you the most about the idea of working with exotic animals as a vet?

CHAPTER 10

Farm Animals and Livestock

Farm animals like cows, sheep, and chickens might seem ordinary, but they play an extraordinary role in our lives. They provide us with food, wool, and so much more. Taking care of them isn't just about feeding and sheltering them— it's about understanding their health and needs to ensure they thrive. For veterinarians who work with farm animals, every day on the job is an adventure. It's a chance to help these hardworking animals stay healthy while also supporting farmers and their communities.

Why Farm Vets Are Important

Farm veterinarians are like detectives, problem-solvers, and health experts all rolled into one. They don't just work with individual animals; they care for entire herds and flocks. Their work helps farmers keep their animals healthy, which is essential for providing milk, eggs, and meat to families around the world.

For example, a vet might visit a dairy farm to check on a cow that isn't producing as much milk as usual. Through a thorough examination, the vet might discover the cow has a condition called mastitis, which is an infection of the udder. The vet would treat the infection and work with the farmer to prevent it from happening again.

Sometimes, vets also help deliver baby animals. Imagine assisting a sheep during the birth of her lambs or helping a cow with a difficult calving. These moments can be challenging, but they're also incredibly rewarding.

Real-Life Stories From the Farm

Dr. Alvarez, a farm vet, once helped save a flock of chickens that had a mysterious illness. The chickens were acting lethargic and weren't laying eggs. After careful observation and testing, Dr. Alvarez discovered they had a vitamin deficiency. She worked with the farmer to adjust their diet, and soon, the chickens were back to clucking happily and laying eggs again.

Another vet, Dr. Patel, works with sheep on large farms. One summer, a heatwave caused many sheep to overheat. Dr. Patel helped the farmer create shaded areas and provided special cooling sprays to keep the sheep comfortable. Her quick thinking saved many animals and taught the farmer how to prepare for future heatwaves.

These stories show how vets not only treat animals but also educate farmers on how to prevent problems. Their work keeps farm animals healthy and ensures farms can continue to operate smoothly.

Surprising Farm Animal Facts

Farm animals have their own quirks that make them fascinating. Did you know that cows have best friends? Studies have shown that cows form strong bonds with certain members of their herd, and being separated from their best friend can stress them out.

Sheep are incredibly intelligent and can recognize faces—both humans and sheep! They have excellent memories and can even remember their flockmates after being apart for years. They're also very social animals and thrive in groups.

Chickens are more complex than they seem. They can recognize over 100 different faces—both human and chicken! They also communicate with each other using a variety of clucks and chirps, and mother hens even "talk" to their chicks before they hatch.

Imagining Your Own Farm Vet Adventure

If you were a farm vet, what kind of animals would you like to work with? Would you visit a sheep farm in the countryside or a bustling dairy farm? Picture yourself examining a calf, helping a chicken recover from an illness, or advising a farmer on the best care for their livestock.

Farm vets are vital to keeping animals healthy, and their work has a ripple effect on communities. By ensuring that farms run smoothly, vets help provide food and resources to people all over the world. It's a challenging but deeply fulfilling career for anyone who loves animals and enjoys problem-solving.

Questions

- What do you think would be the most exciting part of being a farm vet, and why?

- How do farm vets help entire communities, not just individual animals?

- Why do you think it's important for vets to educate farmers about animal care?

- What surprised you the most about the stories or facts shared in this chapter?

- If you could visit a farm to see a vet in action, what animal or situation would you want to learn about?

PART 3

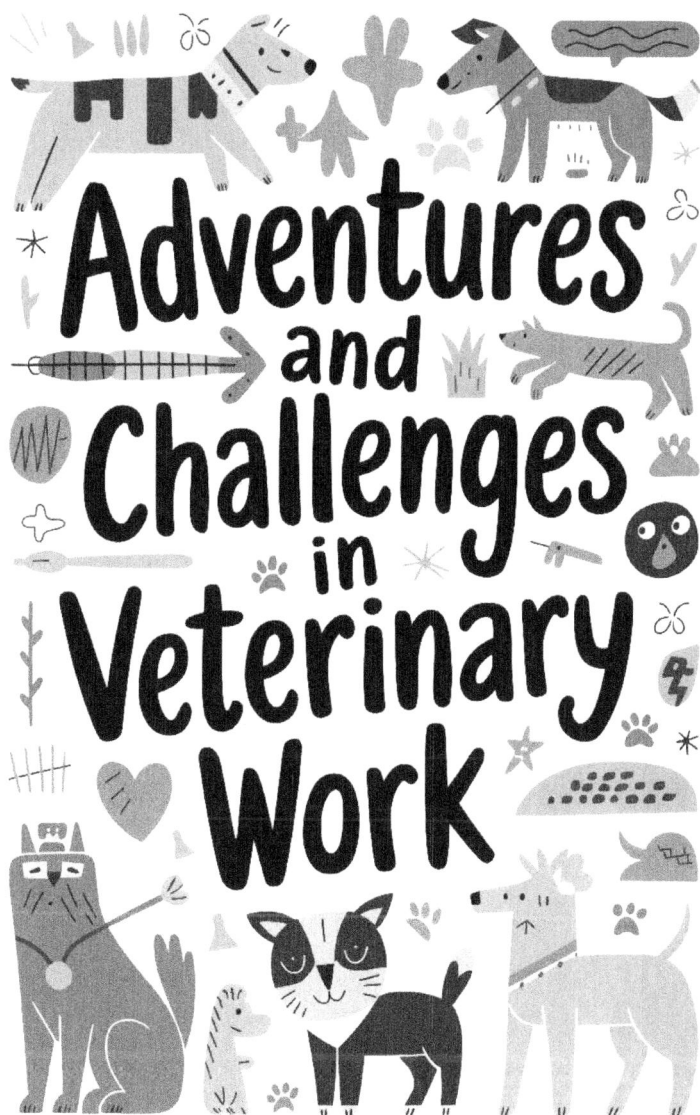

Adventures and Challenges in Veterinary Work

CHAPTER 11

The Science Behind Treating Animals

A Vet's Secret Weapon: Science

Imagine you're a detective, but instead of solving human mysteries, your cases involve animals that can't tell you what's wrong. That's what veterinarians do every day! They use science to uncover clues and figure out how to help. When an animal isn't feeling well, vets rely on tools like X-rays, blood tests, and microscopes to reveal the answers hidden inside the body.

Take Milo, a playful dog who suddenly starts limping. His owner notices he isn't his usual energetic self and takes him to the vet. The vet first looks at Milo's paw, thinking maybe he stepped on something sharp. When that doesn't explain the problem, the vet uses an X-ray machine. The X-ray shows a tiny crack in Milo's bone—something invisible to the naked eye. With this information, the vet puts Milo's leg in a cast and gives him medicine to help with the pain. Using the science of X-rays, Milo is on the road to recovery.

Science also helps vets identify illnesses. Imagine a cat named Bella who seems tired all the time and isn't eating. The vet takes a small sample of Bella's blood and runs a test to check for infections or organ problems. The results reveal that Bella has a low red blood cell count, a condition called anemia. With this knowledge, the vet gives Bella a special diet and medication to boost her health.

Amazing Tools of the Trade

Veterinary science has some fascinating tools. X-rays and ultrasounds let vets see what's happening inside an animal's body without surgery. For example, ultrasounds use sound waves to create pictures of organs like the heart or kidneys, which can help diagnose serious problems.

Microscopes are another essential tool. When a vet suspects that a dog might have parasites like fleas or ticks, they might use a microscope to confirm their suspicions. This tiny world reveals the culprits behind itching or illness and helps the vet choose the right treatment.

One especially cool tool is the endoscope, which is like a tiny camera on a flexible tube. Vets can use it to look inside an animal's stomach or throat. Imagine a parrot named Kiwi who swallows a shiny coin by mistake. The endoscope allows the vet to carefully remove the coin without needing surgery, saving Kiwi from a dangerous situation.

Real-Life Success Stories

Vets see the magic of science in action every day. Ruby, a golden retriever, couldn't run or play because her back legs hurt. An X-ray revealed arthritis, a condition that makes joints stiff. With the help of medicine and physical therapy, Ruby is now able to chase her favorite ball again.

In another case, a tiny hamster named Chip started losing patches of fur. His owner brought him to the vet, who used a microscope to find tiny mites on his skin. After a few treatments, Chip's fur grew back, and he was his happy, wiggly self again.

Be a Vet Detective

Want to try solving an animal mystery? Create your own "animal medical chart."

Start by imagining a pretend pet—maybe a dog named Max or a rabbit named Hazel. Write down some symptoms, like "not eating" or "scratching a lot." Then, decide which scientific tools you'd use to solve the case. Would you choose an X-ray, a blood test, or a microscope?

Vets combine science with compassion to help animals heal. Whether they're treating a playful puppy or a tired turtle, their work shows just how powerful science can be when it's used to care for others.

Questions

- How do vets use science to solve health mysteries for animals?

- What tools do vets rely on to understand what's happening inside an animal's body?

- Can you think of an example where science helped save an animal's life?

- If you were a vet, which tool would you want to use most and why?

- Why do you think understanding science is important for helping animals?

CHAPTER 12

Wildlife and Conservation Vets

Heroes for Wild Animals

When you think of veterinarians, you might picture them helping dogs, cats, or farm animals. But some vets dedicate their lives to wildlife, working with creatures that roam the forests, swim in the oceans, or soar in the skies. Wildlife and conservation vets are like superheroes for animals in the wild. Their work helps protect endangered species and keeps ecosystems in balance.

Imagine you're a vet called to help a sea turtle found tangled in plastic. The turtle has a cracked shell and trouble swimming. A wildlife vet carefully removes the plastic, cleans the wounds, and applies a special resin to repair the shell. After weeks of care and monitoring, the turtle is released back into the ocean, ready to swim free once again.

These vets also work to prevent problems before they happen. They might vaccinate wild animals to stop the spread of diseases or track herds of elephants to ensure they have enough space and food to thrive. Their work takes them to jungles, mountains, deserts, and beyond.

Amazing Wildlife Rescue Stories

In Africa, a wildlife vet named Dr. Kalembe once saved a young elephant that fell into a muddy well. The calf was stuck and couldn't move. Dr. Kalembe and her team used ropes, pulleys, and plenty of teamwork to pull the elephant out. Once free, the vet treated the calf for cuts and dehydration. Soon, the baby elephant was reunited with its herd—a heartwarming success!

In Australia, Dr. Nguyen, a vet who specializes in koalas, helped during wildfires that left many animals injured. She treated burns, provided food, and helped release koalas back into safe habitats. Her work not only saved individual animals but also gave hope to communities devastated by the fires.

How Kids Can Help Wildlife

You don't need to be a vet to make a difference for wildlife. Small actions can help protect animals and the planet. For example, building a bird feeder in your backyard provides food for local birds, especially during colder months. Reducing plastic waste by using reusable bags and bottles keeps trash out of oceans, where it can harm marine life.

If you live near a park or forest, picking up litter during a family hike helps create a safer space for animals. Even learning about endangered species and sharing what you know with friends can raise awareness and inspire others to help.

An Adventure Across the Globe

Wildlife conservation happens everywhere. Picture a map of the world dotted with amazing projects:

- In India, vets work to protect Bengal tigers, using GPS collars to track their movements and keep them safe from poachers.

- In the Amazon rainforest, vets care for rescued sloths and monkeys who have lost their homes due to deforestation.

- In the Arctic, teams help polar bears struggling with shrinking sea ice by studying their behavior and finding ways to protect their habitats.

Each project is like a puzzle piece, coming together to form a bigger picture of wildlife conservation.

Be a Wildlife Hero

Want to imagine yourself as a wildlife vet? Pretend you're treating a penguin with an injured wing. What tools would you use? How would you help the penguin get better and return to its icy home? Write down your ideas and share them with a friend or family member.

Wildlife and conservation vets show us how important it is to care for all creatures, great and small. By protecting wildlife, they're also protecting the planet we all share.

Questions

- Why is the work of wildlife and conservation vets important for animals and the environment?

- What do you think would be the most challenging part of helping wild animals?

- How can small actions, like reducing waste or building bird feeders, make a big difference?

- If you were a wildlife vet, which animal would you want to help most and why?

- What surprised you about the stories or global conservation projects shared in this chapter?

CHAPTER 13

The Challenges of Being a Vet

The Tough Side of the Job

Being a veterinarian is one of the most rewarding jobs in the world, but it's also one of the most challenging. While vets love helping animals, they sometimes face tough situations that test their skills and emotions. Whether it's dealing with a sick pet, managing a tricky surgery, or comforting an owner, vets need to stay strong, calm and focused.

Imagine being a vet called to help a horse named Bella who isn't eating or moving well. Bella's owner is worried, and the vet has to act quickly. After examining Bella, the vet discovers she has colic, a serious stomach problem that can be life-threatening. The vet performs an emergency treatment to relieve Bella's pain. Even though it's a long, exhausting process, the vet is determined to help Bella recover—and in the end, Bella's life is saved.

Sometimes, the challenges aren't just about the animals. Vets also work with people, like pet owners or farmers, who may be anxious or upset. A vet needs to explain what's happening and help them make the best decisions for their animals, even when the situation is difficult.

Handling Emotions and Staying Resilient

Because vets care deeply about animals, it's hard for them when things don't go as planned. They might feel sad if they can't save a beloved pet or stressed when faced with a tough decision. To handle these emotions, vets learn to stay resilient—meaning they find ways to keep going, even when things are hard.

One way vets stay resilient is by focusing on the good moments. For every tough case, there are many happy ones, like seeing a puppy recover from an illness or a rescued sea turtle swimming free again. Vets also support each other, sharing stories and advice to stay strong as a team.

Problem-Solving Like a Vet

Want to experience some of the challenges vets face? Imagine this scenario: You're a vet, and a farmer brings in a sheep that isn't eating and seems weak. What do you do?

First, you'd gather clues by asking questions: When did the sheep start feeling sick? Is anyone else in the flock acting strangely? Then, you'd examine the sheep, looking for signs like a fever or unusual behavior. Finally, you'd decide on a plan—maybe treating the sheep with medicine and checking the rest of the flock to make sure they're healthy.

By thinking like a vet, you can practice problem-solving and develop skills to handle tricky situations.

The Rewards Outweigh the Challenges

Even though being a vet can be tough, the rewards make it all worthwhile. Vets get to see animals heal, build trust with their owners, and make a real difference in their communities. Whether they're saving a kitten stuck in a tree, helping a cow deliver a calf, or performing life-saving surgery, vets know their work matters.

Questions

- Why do you think it's important for vets to stay calm and focused during tough situations?

- What emotions might a vet feel when dealing with a difficult case, and how can they handle those feelings?

- If you were a vet, how would you comfort an anxious pet owner?

- What's one example of how problem-solving helps vets overcome challenges?

- Why do you think many vets say their job is rewarding, even with the challenges they face?

CHAPTER 14

Working as a Team

A Day in the Life of a Veterinary Team

Behind every veterinarian is a team of skilled, hardworking people who make everything run smoothly. When you visit an animal clinic, it's not just the vet who helps your pet. Vet nurses, technicians, receptionists, and even specialists all play important roles. Together, they form a team that works like a well-oiled machine to help animals feel better.

Picture a dog named Daisy who comes to the clinic for surgery. While the vet operates, a vet technician monitors

Daisy's heart rate and breathing. A veterinary nurse prepares medicines and comforts Daisy as she wakes up. Meanwhile, the receptionist talks with Daisy's owner, answering questions and scheduling follow-up care. Everyone works together to ensure Daisy has the best possible experience.

Teamwork is essential, whether it's a bustling animal clinic, a farm visit, or a wildlife rescue. No one can do it all alone, and when each person contributes their unique skills, amazing things happen.

Meet the Team

Each person on a veterinary team has a special job:

- Veterinarian: The leader of the team, vets diagnose illnesses, perform surgeries, and create treatment plans.

- Vet Technicians: These animal care experts assist with exams, run lab tests, and help during surgeries.

- Vet Nurses: Think of them as animal nurses! They provide treatments, comfort animals, and educate owners.

- Receptionists: They're the friendly faces who greet owners, schedule appointments, and handle paperwork.

- Specialists: These vets focus on specific areas, like surgery, dentistry, or exotic animals.

Each role is important, and when everyone works together, they can handle anything from a kitten's first check-up to an emergency operation.

Learning Teamwork in Your Own Life

Teamwork isn't just for veterinary clinics—it's a skill you can practice every day. Think about when you play a sport, work on a group project at school, or even do chores with your family. Teamwork means listening to others, sharing ideas, and helping each other reach a goal.

For example, if you're building a treehouse with friends, one person might design the plan, another might gather materials, and someone else might hammer the nails. By dividing the work and cooperating, you'll finish faster—and have more fun along the way!

A Teamwork Challenge

Ready to put your teamwork skills to the test? Imagine you're part of a veterinary team helping a sick parrot named Mango. The parrot needs medicine and a new diet, but he's nervous around people. How would you work with your team to help Mango feel safe and comfortable? Maybe one person distracts Mango with a treat while another gently administers the medicine. Think about how each team member can play a role in Mango's care.

Why Teamwork Matters

Good teamwork makes the job easier and helps animals feel better faster. For vets, teamwork means knowing they're never alone, even during the toughest cases. Everyone on the team shares the same goal: giving animals the best care possible.

When you work as part of a team, you also learn from others. A vet might teach a technician a new skill, or a nurse might share tips with an owner on comforting their pet. This exchange of knowledge helps everyone grow.

Whether it's helping animals or solving problems at school, teamwork brings people together and proves that amazing things happen when everyone works toward the same goal.

Questions

- What are some ways teamwork helps vets care for animals more effectively?

- Which role in a veterinary team sounds the most interesting to you, and why?

- Can you think of a time when you worked on a team? What made it successful?

- Why is it important for team members to share their unique skills?

- If you were helping a nervous animal like Mango, what role would you want to play on the team?

CHAPTER 15

Fun and Rewarding Parts of the Job

Being a veterinarian is an incredible journey full of moments that make all the hard work worthwhile. Every day, vets have the chance to make a real difference in the lives of animals and their families. From saving lives to spreading knowledge, the job is as rewarding as it is challenging. Let's dive into the heartwarming parts of this amazing profession.

Heartwarming Stories of Reunions

One of the most special moments for any vet is seeing an animal reunited with its family after recovering from an illness or injury. Dr. Sanders, a small-animal vet, once treated a mischievous golden retriever named Max. Max had swallowed an entire sock, leaving him in pain and unable to eat. Dr. Sanders performed surgery to remove the sock and carefully monitored Max during his recovery. When Max's family came to pick him up, his joyful bark and wagging tail brought tears to their eyes. For Dr. Sanders, seeing Max healthy and his family so grateful was an unforgettable moment.

In another instance, Dr. Alvarez, a farm vet, worked with a family whose sheepdog, Daisy, had suffered a leg injury. With careful treatment, Daisy was soon back on her feet, running alongside her flock. The family was so relieved to see Daisy happy and active again. Moments like these remind vets why their work is so meaningful—they're not just helping animals; they're strengthening bonds between animals and their humans.

The Joy of Helping Animals Heal

There's a unique joy in watching an animal regain its health and happiness. Dr. Nguyen, a wildlife vet, once treated a hawk with a broken wing. After weeks of care, the hawk was ready to return to the wild. Watching it spread its wings and soar into the sky was a powerful reminder of the impact vets can have on the lives of animals.

Even in everyday situations, vets experience the joy of recovery. Dr. Patel, who works with farm animals, recalls helping a lamb that had trouble walking due to a joint infection. After treatment and plenty of rest, the lamb was hopping around the pasture again, much to the delight of its owners.

Teaching and Educating

Another rewarding part of the job is teaching people how to care for their animals. Sometimes, pet owners don't know how much care their animals need, and vets can step in as educators. Dr. Patel once worked with a family that was new to raising sheep. She helped them set up a feeding schedule, taught them how to spot signs of illness, and showed them the best way to keep their flock healthy. Over time, the family became confident shepherds, supported by Dr. Patel's expertise.

Vets also teach kids how to care for their pets. Imagine a vet showing a group of students how to brush a dog's teeth or explaining why regular check-ups are so important. By educating others, vets are ensuring animals receive better care everywhere.

A "Thank You, Vet!" Activity

Have you ever thought about how much work vets do to keep animals healthy and happy? Take a moment to show your appreciation! Create a "Thank You, Vet!" card or drawing. Maybe you want to thank a vet for saving your pet or simply let them know how much you admire their work. These small gestures mean a lot to the people who dedicate their lives to helping animals.

Celebrating the Rewards of Veterinary Work

Being a vet isn't just about medical treatments— It's about fostering an environment where animals and humans thrive together. Every happy wag of a tail, every purr, and every chirp is a reminder of the incredible impact vets have on the world. It's a job that brings joy not only to animals but also to their families and communities.

Questions

- What do you think is the most rewarding part of being a vet, and why?

- How does helping animals also bring happiness to their owners?

- Why is educating pet owners such an important part of a vet's job?

- Can you think of a time when you helped an animal or pet? How did it make you feel?

- If you were a vet, how would you celebrate the animals you helped recover?

PART 4

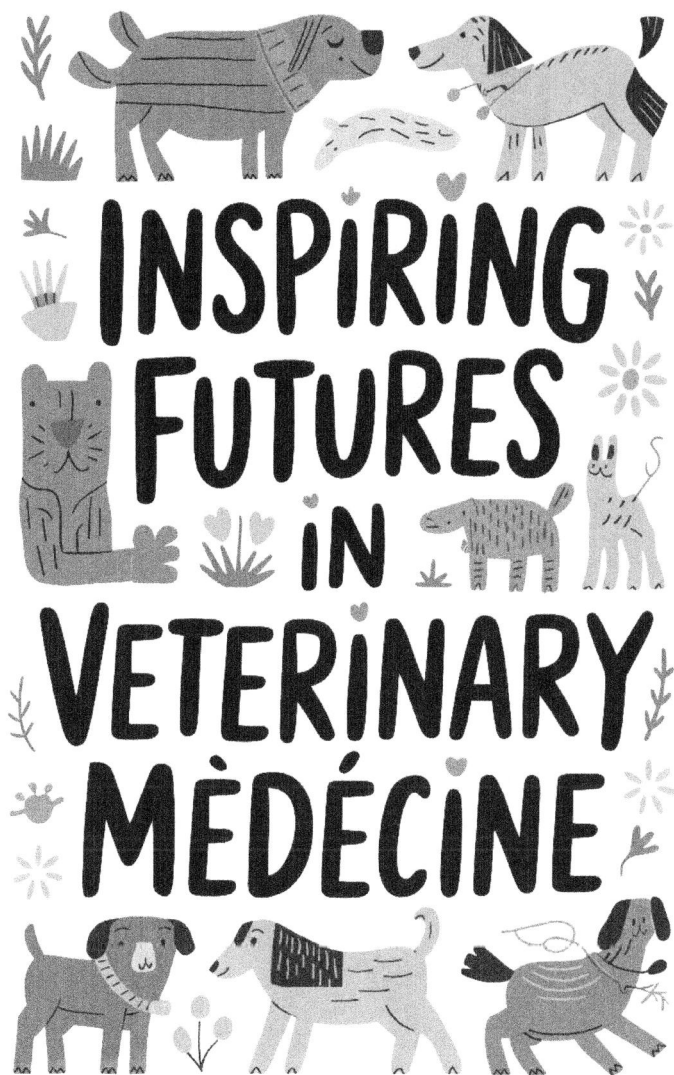

INSPIRING FUTURES iN VETERINARY MÈDÉCINE

CHAPTER 16

Tips for Kids Who Love Animals

If you're someone who loves animals and dreams of becoming a vet one day, you're already on the right path! Vets spend their lives working with animals, but you can start right now, learning more and taking care of creatures, big or small. There are many ways you can explore your love for animals, whether through fun activities, hobbies, or helping those in need. Here's how you can get started on your own animal adventure!

Start a Pet Journal

One of the best ways to begin learning about animals is by observing them. Whether you have a pet at home or just love watching animals in your yard, starting a pet journal is a fantastic way to keep track of what you see. A pet journal allows you to record details about animals—how they behave, what they eat, how they play, and even how they interact with other animals. You can draw pictures, take notes, or even write stories about your experiences.

Imagine you're a vet, and your job is to keep track of how a pet is doing. A vet might take notes about how an animal is behaving to help diagnose if something is wrong. By doing this in your journal, you'll start thinking like a vet. You'll learn how to pay attention to small changes in behavior, which is an important skill for anyone who loves animals.

Volunteer at Animal Shelters

Another great way to get involved is by volunteering at a local animal shelter. Shelters are places where animals wait for a new home, and they often need help from caring people like you. You might get to walk dogs, clean cages, feed the animals or help with other important tasks. As a volunteer, you'll learn how to handle different animals and understand their needs. It's a way to get hands-on experience and practice the skills that vets use every day.

At the shelter, you might meet veterinarians and see how they care for animals. Watching a vet in action will show you what it takes to help animals stay healthy. You might even have the chance to learn about animal care practices, such as how to check for signs of illness, treat injuries, and perform check-ups. Volunteering gives you a behind-the-scenes look at what it takes to help animals in need.

Make Simple Items for Animals

Being a future vet is all about showing animals that you care, and sometimes, the simplest acts of kindness can make a big difference. One fun and easy way to help animals is by making items for them, like pet toys or birdhouses. You can build a birdhouse out of wood and hang it in your yard. Watching birds fly in and out of their new home is a great way to observe wildlife. You could even start a small bird-watching journal, writing down what types of birds you see.

You can also make pet toys for animals at the shelter or for your own pets. A simple rope toy for a dog or a homemade scratching post for a cat is not only fun to make, but it also provides comfort and entertainment to animals. You might not realize it, but by creating something for an animal, you're helping improve their well-being. This is something that vets think about all the time. They know how important it is to keep animals happy and comfortable while they are being treated or waiting for a home.

Visit Your Local Library or Shelter

If you want to learn more about animals, visiting your local library is a great place to start. Libraries are full of books about animals, veterinary science, and ways to care for pets. You can read up on animal species, learn about the history of veterinary medicine, or explore how animals communicate and interact. Libraries also often have special programs, workshops, or events where you can meet experts and learn even more.

Another place to visit is your local animal shelter. Not only will you get to see the animals, but many shelters offer tours or educational programs where you can learn about the work they do. Some shelters even allow kids to shadow the staff or join special youth programs. These experiences help you build empathy for animals, which is a key trait for any future vet. You might even get to participate in special fundraisers to help animals in need!

Questions

- What animals do you enjoy observing the most, and what have you learned about their behavior?

- How do you think volunteering at an animal shelter can help you learn more about being a vet?

- What's one item you could make for an animal that would improve their comfort or happiness?

- How can visiting a library or shelter help you in your journey to becoming a vet?

- What qualities do you think a vet must have to work well with animals, and how can you practice these qualities at home or school?

CHAPTER 17

Cool Animal Careers Besides Being a Vet

When you think about working with animals, the first job that might come to mind is being a veterinarian. But did you know there are many other amazing careers that allow you to work with animals and help them in unique ways? These careers are just as important to animal welfare, and each one offers something different. Let's take a closer look at some of these cool animal-related careers.

Marine Biologist

If you've ever wondered what life is like under the sea, a career as a marine biologist could be perfect for you. Marine biologists study ocean animals like whales, dolphins, sharks, and even tiny creatures like plankton. They explore how these animals live, what they need to survive, and how we can protect them from pollution and other threats.

Marine biologists work both in the lab and out in the field. Sometimes, they dive into the ocean to study marine life up close, while other times, they may study animals from the shore or aboard research vessels. They collect data on ocean ecosystems, and their work helps to ensure that we can continue to enjoy and protect the ocean's diverse creatures.

Veterinarians and marine biologists often work together when it comes to the health of marine animals. If a whale or sea turtle is sick or injured, both marine biologists and vets play crucial roles in treating them and making sure they recover. Marine biologists help identify the problem in the animal's environment, while vets provide medical care.

Zookeeper

Have you ever wondered how the animals in a zoo are cared for? That's where zookeepers come in! Zookeepers are responsible for the day-to-day care of the animals in their charge. They feed the animals, clean their enclosures, and make sure they're healthy and comfortable. Zookeepers also observe the animals closely, looking for signs of illness or distress.

Although being a zookeeper isn't the same as being a vet, the two careers often go hand in hand. Zookeepers work closely with veterinarians to monitor the health of zoo animals. If an animal is sick or hurt, it's the zookeeper's job to alert the vet, who then provides treatment. Zookeepers also help educate the public about animal care and conservation efforts, making them an essential part of animal welfare.

Wildlife Conservationist

Wildlife conservationists are dedicated to protecting animals and their habitats. They work in the wild, in reserves, and in natural parks to monitor and protect endangered species. Their goal is to ensure that animals like elephants, tigers, and polar bears have the space and resources they need to thrive.

Conservationists may conduct research, restore damaged ecosystems, or create laws and policies to protect wildlife. Some focus on protecting a specific species, while others work to preserve entire ecosystems. They often collaborate with veterinarians to monitor the health of wildlife populations, especially in protected areas. By working together, vets and wildlife conservationists ensure that animals remain safe and healthy in their natural environments.

Animal Behaviorist

Do you love watching animals and figuring out how they think and behave? Animal behaviorists do just that! They study how animals interact with their environment, with other animals, and with humans. They work to understand why animals behave the way they do and how they can be trained or helped to change certain behaviors.

For example, if a dog is acting out by chewing furniture or barking excessively, an animal behaviorist might step in to figure out why the dog is acting this way. They then create strategies to help the dog learn new, healthier behaviors. Animal behaviorists can work with a wide variety of animals, from pets to wild animals, and they often team up with vets to create comprehensive care plans.

Quiz: "Which Animal Career Is Perfect for You?"

Now it's your turn to discover which animal career might be perfect for you! Take this fun quiz to find out which job you'd enjoy the most.

1. What do you love doing most in your free time?

a) Exploring nature

b) Watching animal documentaries

c) Visiting zoos or wildlife parks

d) Observing animals at home or at the shelter

2. How do you feel about working outdoors?

a) I love it! I'm always up for an adventure.

b) I enjoy it sometimes, but I also like being inside.

c) I prefer staying indoors, where it's cozy.

d) I'd like a balance of both!

3.   What do you want to learn more about?

a) Ocean animals and their habitats

b) How to care for animals in a zoo or sanctuary

c) How to protect wildlife and their environments

d) Animal behavior and how they communicate

4.   Which animal would you love to work with most?

a) Dolphins and whales

b) Tigers, elephants, and monkeys

c) Endangered species like pandas or rhinos

d) Dogs, cats, or exotic pets

How Different Roles Contribute to Animal Welfare

Each of these careers contributes in its own special way to the welfare of animals. Marine biologists protect ocean life and study the effects of pollution, ensuring that aquatic animals have healthy environments. Zookeepers ensure that zoo animals receive proper care and attention, while wildlife conservationists protect habitats and fight to save endangered species. Animal behaviorists work to improve animals' relationships with humans, making them healthier and happier.

All of these professionals play a role in the well-being of animals, and in many cases, they work alongside veterinarians to keep animals safe and healthy. Vets rely on the research and care provided by marine biologists, conservationists, zookeepers, and behaviorists to make the best decisions for animal health. Whether you become a vet or choose another animal-related career, you'll be helping animals live better lives.

Questions

- Which animal career do you think would be the most exciting and why?

- How do you think marine biologists and veterinarians work together to help sea animals?

- What role do zookeepers play in keeping zoo animals safe, and how might their work connect to veterinary care?

- How can understanding animal behavior help improve the way we care for animals?

- How do you think working as a wildlife conservationist can help protect endangered species and their habitats?

CHAPTER 18

Inspiring Stories of Real Vets

Veterinarians play a crucial role in the well-being of animals all around the world. They not only provide medical care, but they also help protect endangered species, assist with animal conservation, and even step in during natural disasters. The following stories showcase real-life vets who have made remarkable contributions to animal welfare. These vets have shown incredible dedication, compassion, and bravery, often overcoming great challenges to make a difference in the lives of animals.

Dr. Thinlay Bhutia: Helping Stray Animals in India

Dr. Thinlay Bhutia, a dedicated veterinarian in Sikkim, India, has made significant strides in managing the state's stray dog population and combating rabies. In 2006, he co-founded the Sikkim Anti-Rabies and Animal Health (SARAH) program, India's first government-sanctioned initiative for statewide rabies and stray dog population control.

Through mass vaccination and sterilization campaigns, the program has effectively reduced rabies cases and humanely managed the stray dog population. Dr. Bhutia's efforts have not only improved animal welfare but also enhanced public health in the region.

Dr. Gladys Kalema-Zikusoka: Protecting Wildlife in Africa

Dr. Gladys Kalema-Zikusoka is a pioneering Ugandan veterinarian and conservationist, renowned for her work in integrating wildlife preservation with public health initiatives. In 1996, she became Uganda's first wildlife veterinary officer, focusing on the health of endangered mountain gorillas in Bwindi Impenetrable National Park. Recognizing the interconnectedness of human and wildlife health, she founded Conservation Through Public Health (CTPH) in 2003. CTPH addresses zoonotic disease transmission by improving healthcare and sanitation in communities adjacent to gorilla habitats, thereby reducing disease risks for both humans and gorillas. Dr. Kalema-Zikusoka's holistic approach has been instrumental in increasing the mountain gorilla population and fostering coexistence between local communities and wildlife.

Her innovative work has earned her numerous accolades, including the United Nations Environment Programme's Champion of the Earth for Science and Innovation in 2021.

Dr. Ben Brown: Helping Animals After Disasters

Dr. Ben Brown, an Australian veterinarian, has been instrumental in providing emergency veterinary care during natural disasters, particularly the devastating bushfires that have impacted Australia's unique wildlife. As a Disaster Response Veterinarian with World Vets, Dr. Brown led a team during the 2019-2020 Australian bushfires, collaborating with local veterinary clinics and organizations to treat injured wildlife, livestock, and domestic animals. His team's efforts included treating animals suffering from burns, smoke inhalation, and other fire-related injuries, providing critical care to species such as koalas, kangaroos, and various bird species.

Dr. Brown's dedication highlights the vital role veterinarians play in disaster response, ensuring the welfare and rehabilitation of animals affected by such catastrophic events.

Dr. Brian Stacy: Saving Sea Turtles in the U.S.

Dr. Brian Stacy is a distinguished veterinarian and scientist with NOAA Fisheries' Office of Protected Resources, specializing in the health and recovery of threatened and endangered sea turtles in the United States. His role encompasses monitoring and investigating causes of sea turtle strandings, assessing human impacts on their populations, and addressing diseases affecting these marine reptiles. Dr. Stacy also plays a pivotal role in planning and responding to environmental crises, such as oil spills and cold-stunning events, which can severely impact sea turtle populations.

Throughout his career, Dr. Stacy has been actively involved in various emergency responses to protect sea turtles. Notably, during the 2010 Deepwater Horizon oil spill, he led efforts to rescue and rehabilitate over 300 oiled sea turtles from affected offshore areas. These turtles were treated, cleaned, and successfully released back into the wild, showcasing his commitment to mitigating human-induced threats to marine life.

Dr. Stacy's work exemplifies the critical role veterinarians play in marine conservation, particularly in addressing the challenges sea turtles face due to environmental hazards and human activities. His dedication to the rehabilitation and recovery of these endangered species highlights the importance of veterinary expertise in wildlife conservation efforts.

Activity: Write Your Own Vet Adventure

Now that you've read about these inspiring vets, it's time for you to get creative. Imagine you are a veterinarian, and you're on an exciting adventure to help an animal in need. You could be working in the wild to save an endangered species, helping animals recover after a disaster, or even discovering a new way to care for animals. Write a short story about your adventure and the challenges you face. What animals do you help? What tools do you need? How do you feel when the animal is saved?

Questions

- Which of these real vet stories inspired you the most and why?

- How do you think Dr. Thinlay Bhutia's work helps improve the lives of stray animals in India?

- What do you think are some of the biggest challenges that Dr. Gladys Kalema-Zikusoka faces when working with wildlife in Africa?

- In what ways do you think Dr. Ben Brown's work after the wildfires can inspire other veterinarians to help during emergencies?

- How can Dr. Brian Stacy's efforts to save sea turtles teach us about the connection between vets and the environment?

CHAPTER 19

The Future of Veterinary Medicine

Veterinary medicine is constantly evolving, and it's amazing to think about how far technology has come in helping veterinarians care for animals. From life-saving surgeries to understanding animals on a molecular level, the future of veterinary care is filled with exciting possibilities. Let's take a look at some of the groundbreaking advancements that are shaping the way vets will work in the future.

Robotic Surgery: Precision at Its Best

One of the most exciting developments is robotic surgery. Imagine a robot that can help a veterinarian perform surgery with incredible precision! While it might sound like science fiction, robotic surgery is already being used in some veterinary clinics. These robots assist vets during complicated procedures, allowing them to perform surgeries with extreme accuracy. The robotic arm can make tiny, exact movements that might be too difficult for a human hand, reducing the risk of mistakes. This technology is especially helpful in surgeries where the area is difficult to reach or when the animal is very small. With robotic surgery, recovery times for animals may also be shorter, allowing them to heal more quickly and get back to playing and running around.

DNA Research: Unlocking the Secrets of Animal Health

Another exciting advancement in veterinary medicine is DNA research. Scientists have discovered that studying an animal's DNA can reveal a lot about its health and future needs. For example, by examining an animal's genes, veterinarians can identify if they are at risk for certain diseases or conditions, even before symptoms appear. This means that vets can catch health problems early and start treatment right away, which can save lives. Additionally, DNA research is helping vets understand more about different animal species and how to care for them properly. This is especially important when it comes to endangered animals, where scientists and vets are working together to protect species from disappearing forever.

Microchips: Helping Pets Find Their Way Home

But technology in veterinary medicine doesn't just stop at surgery and DNA. There are other incredible innovations, like microchips, which are small devices that can be placed under an animal's skin. These chips are used to help track pets if they get lost. The chip contains a tiny piece of information about the animal, such as its name and the contact details of the owner. When a lost animal is found, a vet or animal shelter can scan the microchip and immediately get the information they need to return the pet home. This simple yet powerful technology has already helped reunite thousands of lost pets with their families. It's a great example of how technology can make a huge difference in the lives of animals and their owners.

What's Next? Imagining the Future of Veterinary Medicine

As exciting as these advancements are, the future of veterinary medicine is still full of possibilities. What other incredible tools will vets have at their disposal? Imagine a world where veterinarians can use virtual reality to practice surgeries before performing them or where they can send animals' medical information to a specialist halfway around the world for advice in real-time. What if future vets could use advanced technology to monitor an animal's health 24/7, making sure they are always in tip-top shape?

There are endless possibilities for the future of veterinary care, and you could be the one to help make them a reality! Who knows? Maybe you'll invent a new piece of technology that changes the way animals are cared for. The future of veterinary medicine is bright, and it's up to the next generation, like you, to dream big and imagine what comes next.

Questions

- How do you think robotic surgery could help veterinarians take better care of animals?

- What do you think veterinarians could learn from studying the DNA of animals?

- Why do you think microchips are such an important tool for veterinarians and pet owners?

- What other technological advancements do you think could be helpful for vets in the future?

- If you could invent a new technology to help animals, what would it be, and how would it work?

CHAPTER 20

Becoming a Vet

A Roadmap to Becoming a Vet

Have you ever wondered what it's like to be a veterinarian? A vet is someone who dedicates their life to helping animals, whether it's through medical treatment, surgeries, or preventive care. Becoming a vet is a rewarding journey, but like any big dream, it takes hard work, dedication, and a passion for animals. If you're interested in becoming a vet, let's break down the path you can take—from school all the way to the veterinary clinic!

The first step in your vet journey is to focus on doing well in school. A solid foundation in subjects like science, math, and reading will help you later on. In middle school, focus on subjects like biology and chemistry, which are the building blocks for understanding animal health. Science projects can also be a fun way to start exploring veterinary medicine. For example, you could create a project to learn more about how animals' bodies work or how veterinarians diagnose diseases. Getting curious about how animals function inside and out will help you get one step closer to your goal.

Once you're in high school, the next step is to take advanced science classes like biology, chemistry, and physics. These subjects will give you the knowledge you need to understand animal biology and how to take care of different species. It's also a good idea to look for opportunities to get hands-on experience with animals. Volunteering at animal shelters, zoos, or veterinary clinics is a great way to start learning more about animals and how to care for them. You can also shadow veterinarians or animal care specialists to see what their daily jobs are like. The more experience you have, the better prepared you'll be for the future.

After high school, it's time to think about college. Becoming a veterinarian requires going to veterinary school, which is a special kind of college that focuses on teaching students how to care for animals. To get into vet school, you'll need to first earn a college degree, usually in a science-related field like biology or animal science. Some colleges even offer pre-veterinary programs that will help you prepare for veterinary school. Keep in mind that vet school is competitive, so maintaining a high GPA and gaining experience with animals is very important.

The veterinary school itself takes several years, typically around four years, and includes both classroom learning and hands-on practice. During this time, you'll learn everything about animal health—from anatomy and physiology to diseases and treatments. You'll also gain skills in surgery, diagnosis, and working with different kinds of animals, from pets to farm animals to exotic wildlife. It's a challenging program, but if you love animals and are determined, it's a great opportunity to become an expert in the field.

Fun Ways to Prepare Now

You don't have to wait until you're older to start preparing to become a vet. There are lots of fun, age-appropriate ways to begin learning and developing skills now. One way to prepare is by starting a science project. Try researching how veterinarians treat different types of animals or how animal diseases are diagnosed and treated. You can also start learning basic first-aid skills. Understanding how to help animals in emergencies can be a useful skill to have, and it's something you can start practicing even as a kid!

Another way to prepare is by observing animals closely. Whether you have pets at home or you're visiting a zoo or animal shelter, take the time to really observe the animals. How do they move? What do they eat? What signs of health or illness can you notice? The more you pay attention to animals' behaviors and needs, the better equipped you'll be when you begin your formal training as a vet.

10 Things You Can Do Today to Start Your Vet Journey

1.   Volunteer at an animal shelter or rescue group.

2.   Read books or watch videos about veterinary medicine.

3.   Learn about different animals and their unique needs.

4.   Start a science project related to animals or animal care.

5.   Shadow a local veterinarian or animal care professional.

6.   Learn about basic animal first-aid and how to help in an emergency.

7.   Take advanced science courses in school.

8.   Join an animal club or 4-H group.

9.   Keep a journal about your experiences with animals.

10.   Dream big and start thinking about what kind of vet you want to be!

Questions

- What subjects do you think are most important to study if you want to become a vet?

- How can volunteering with animals help you on your journey to becoming a veterinarian?

- What kind of animals would you like to work with as a vet?

- Why do you think it's important to gain hands-on experience before going to vet school?

- What's one thing you can do today to start preparing for your future as a vet?

EPILOGUE

As you turn the final pages of this book, take a moment to imagine all the incredible possibilities that exist in the world of veterinary medicine. Whether it's helping a beloved pet feel better, rescuing injured wildlife, or discovering new ways to keep animals healthy, the role of a veterinarian is full of adventure, challenge, and heartwarming moments.

By now, you've explored the history of veterinary medicine, met real-life heroes who have dedicated their lives to animals, and even tested your own knowledge with fun activities. You've learned that being a vet is more than just taking care of sick animals—it's about problem solving, compassion, teamwork, and sometimes even a bit of detective work. The best veterinarians are not only skilled but also deeply curious. They ask questions, search for solutions, and never stop learning.

But here's the most exciting part: the future of veterinary medicine is still being written. Maybe one day, new breakthroughs will allow vets to cure diseases that are currently untreatable. Maybe technology will create new ways for vets to communicate with animals. Maybe someone—maybe even you—will invent a new tool that changes the way animals are cared for forever.

Even if you don't become a veterinarian, there are so many ways you can help animals. You might volunteer at an animal shelter, learn how to take care of pets, or even teach others about the importance of wildlife conservation. Every small action matters. A simple act of kindness, like helping an injured bird or making sure a pet has fresh water, can make a world of difference.

So, as you close this book, think about what you've learned and how it might shape your own journey. What part of veterinary medicine fascinated you the most? What questions do you still have? What kind of world do you want to help create for animals in the future? The answers are yours to explore, and the possibilities are endless.

The world of veterinary medicine is waiting for the next generation of animal champions. Whether you follow this path as a career or simply as someone who cares deeply about animals, you have the power to make a difference. Keep asking questions, keep exploring, and never stop being curious about the amazing creatures we share this planet with.